PALEO DIET

PALEOLITHIC NUTRITION - HEALTH FROM NATURE

SUSAN MARGRET WIMMER

ISBN 978-1-63957-055-3

Contents

Preface

This book is about Paleo diet, a dietary method which was used about thousands of years ago. Now, this diet is recognized as healthiest of all. The information in this book focus on promoting this diet - Paleo and also on supplying all the necessary information to the readers who are still thinking about whether to start a Paleo diet or not.

This book will help even the Paleo lovers to find out the scientific basis behind what they are practically doing. I hope this book will be a great source for you to know all that you don't know about Paleo diets and the added few Paleo recipes will definitely be a great start for the new ones!

Happy Paleo Diet!

ONE
WHAT IS A PALEO DIET?

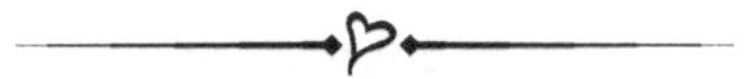

Paleo diet – sounds familiar? Yes, it is. This special diet has been one of the top topics which many nutritionists and health lovers have talked in the past few years. But, I can be sure that it is no more limited to words and many people around the world have started this diet and keep on encouraging others as well. Now, what is this Paleo diet?

Paleo diet is one of the healthiest natural diets, which helps you to remain healthy, strong and energetic. This is the only nutritional approach that guarantees to work with your genetics to stay lean and to reduce those extra fats. Modern researches have proved that our modern diet is full of refined foods, sugars, processed foods and trans fats and these constituents of food has been the culprit causing many diseases such as heart diseases, diabetes, strokes, infertility, liver diseases, depression, cancer, obesity, Alzheimer's and many others.

When a person suddenly checks the list of food which is allowed in a Paleo diet, they show a small hesitation and that is just because they are new to this and have no idea how tasty the Paleo dishes can be. My simple answer to those people is – what about BBQ? You hate that too?

Of course you don't get ice-creams, cookies, cakes, burgers and chips. But, you get a lot healthier foods, which taste great, if you know to cook it right. Paleo diet is a diet based on the foods, which scientists believe that Paleolithic humans might likely have eaten. The foods that are included in this diet contain all natural foods like fresh vegetables, fruits, greens, nuts, meat, fish and etc. But, this diet excludes dairy products and milk, as they were introduced to the diet in very later years. Eliminating all kinds of processed, refined foods and other food additives makes this diet a healthy and friendlier for the digestive system of human beings.

Do you know anything about Paleolithic era? This was an era which lasted about 2.5 million years and according to the historical proofs, this era has ended about 10,000 years ago. When this era has ended, there has been a huge rise in the field of agriculture. Anyhow, it is so amazing how people, who lived 10,000 years ago made wise choices in their diet and we, living in the 21stcentury – very much modern and developed world keeps on adding easy, instant, yet very unhealthy dietary choices into our daily diets. I am pretty sure that we should think twice, the next time we prepare our meal.

Paleo says no to grains and legumes as well. It is because many scientists believe that they were not used by Paleolithic living beings. This has been one of the controversies as some think that there was proof which shows the use of grains and legumes were present in the Paleolithic era. Anyway, the modern Paleo diet, says a strict no to legumes and grains as well.

TWO
MEDICAL BASICS BEHIND

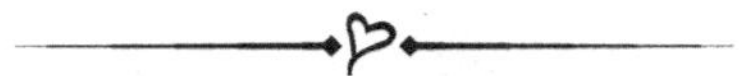

Once you read how the Paleo diet helps the functions of your body, you will definitely realize that it is the best diet in the world.

Even though many people believe that human bodies are the best machines and that whatever they put inside are the best machines and that whatever they put inside are well metabolized, this idea is completely wrong. Many people live their whole life without knowing that their bodies suffered just because they forced their bodies with all the junk.

The metabolic syndrome is one of the major outcomes of all the non-metabolizing things which we add into our system. The percentages of people with metabolic syndromes keep on increasing every day and do you still think that you eat right?

You do not need to believe the words of another person, but, I prefer you see the change yourself. To see and feel the healthy changes of your body, you need to follow the Paleo diet at least for about one month. This diet can literally change your life.

Now let us see how the Paleo diet helps our human body to remain healthy;

1. Paleo diet gives healthy cells

The paleo diet has a good balance between the bad fats and good fats and also it has an enormous amount of omega 3 fats. It is not a secret that our cells are done with a great amount of fats forming its main structures. Maintaining the correct balance of saturated and unsaturated fats helps the cells maintain their structural and functional balance as well.

Moreover, Omega 3 is a main component of bad fats reduction. Omega 3 supplements are now widely recommended as it supports reducing bad fats, preventing heart diseases and also preventing inflammatory diseases of the joints.

2. Healthy Brain

The fishes in the Paleo diet contain omega 3 in great amounts. Omega 3 is very important for the development of the brain and for its functions. That is why the Paleo diet is even recommended for growing teenagers and young adults as well.

3. Less fat and more muscle

A person can increase his weight by increasing the muscle weight or by increasing the fat weight. But, the latter is not a wise option and also it makes the body go out of the shape while making you sick and unhealthy.

In a Paleo diet people increase their muscular weight as the muscles well due to the enough amounts of proteins in the diet. The fats reduce at the same time as there are less fats and low sugars.

More muscles and less fat – what else do you want to get the most good looking body with a good health.

4. Better gut health

Sugars, fats and processed foods can result in gut inflammation and when these kinds of food are combined with the stress of your body, it can totally change your metabolism. The chemical components called as inflammatory cytokines that are produced within the gut may promote these metabolic dysfunctions making the human body sick.

5. Vitamin and mineral blasts

Paleo diets contain a large amount of fruits and veggies and we all know that they are the primary sources of many vitamins and minerals. These vitamins and minerals are essential in healthy metabolic activity of the human body. Adding them in enough amounts helps our body remain healthy, fit and young.

The vitamins boost immunity and thereby prevents from catching infections. They maintain healthy skin, nails and hair of the body and also the bones and teeth. I prefer taking these vitamins and minerals from natural sources through diet than getting it as a supplement.

6. Antioxidants!

Are you an antioxidant hunter? Then here is the best diet. Rather than running behind all kinds of anti-oxidant supplements, it is better that you take it in the natural way.

Antioxidants are responsible in keeping the body young and healthy and also in saving the cells from the metabolic damages by free radicals. It's almost like a disintoxication process. The more you take antioxidants, the more you save yourself!

7. Limits fructose

The Paleo diet recognizes that the human body digests fructose differently than other carbs. Hence, the Paleo diet suggests limiting and strategically choosing the perfect fruit for the job!

Skip the banana and eat a kiwi instead!

8. Better digestion and better absorption

The vegetables and fruits as well as the meat and fishes, are better digested and also well absorbed than the all those processed foods with a lot of food additives. That is why the risk of having any bowel diseases is reduced in the Paleo diet in a great number of folds.

9. Fewer allergies

The dairy products, grains and processed food have a higher incidence of causing allergies among many people. The Paleo diet prohibits these allergenic foods and thereby, we can assure the incidence of getting an allergic reaction is less when you are on a Paleo diet.

10. Increases insulin sensitivity

When you constantly feed your body with sugary foods your body desensitizes to them because it doesn't want or need them anymore. Your body only needs a certain amount of energy, and when you reach that threshold, your cells reject the fuel and store it as fat. If this happens for too long, you will develop insulin insensitivity which means your body will be incapable of recognizing them when your cells are full or not.

Even short-term consumption of a Palaeolithic-type diet improves BP and glucose tolerance, decreases insulin secretion, increases insulin sensitivity and improves lipid profiles without weight loss in healthy sedentary humans.

THREE
SCIENTIFIC FINDINGS

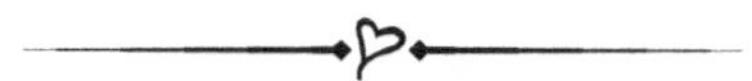

As much as we are concerned about Paleo diet, the scientists are curious too and wanted to find out the real truth hidden inside. Here are some highlights from recent researches:

1. The study, published in the European Journal of Clinical Nutrition, says that Paleo diet can help eliminate fat belly, actually leads to a reduction in triglyceride levels after 6-12 months. The study was conducted on 70 overweight women. But also there was a problem as people did not adhere to such a plan continuously and hence, the affectivity of the research went down later.

2. Another study conducted on 10 healthy women showed a positive effect on the health. These women ate according to the Paleo diet for 5 weeks, not limiting itself to the amount of food and its caloric content. What was the result? Women on average consume fewer calories than usual; they lost weight, normalized diastolic ad systolic blood pressure. Reduced fasting glucose level

and also cholesterol and triglycerides decreased.

3. Another study examines the effect of 10 days of the Paleo diet on human health. Though the subjects lost weight and did not, the researchers concluded that even short-term use of the Paleo diet improves blood pressure and glucose tolerance and reduces insulin and improves the lipid profile.

4. An earlier study examined the relationship between the Mediterranean and the Paleo diet and glucose tolerance. Impaired glucose tolerance, which increases the risk of cardiovascular disease, suppressed better while using Paleo diet. Also, people, adhere to the Paleo diet were able to lose more weight loss.

5. In 2009, a similar result has been shown in randomized trials. 13 diabetic instruction scientists continued a Paleo diet consisting of meat, fish, fruit, vegetables, eggs and nuts, for 3 months. The results are similar to previous studies, the researchers noted that the Paleo diet allows better control of blood sugar levels, and somewhat reduces the risk of cardiovascular disease in type 2 diabetics.

Science never lies. These researches have one thing in common and that is that the Paleo diet has positive effects on our body. When you summarize these studies, it is clear to anyone that the Paleo diet can be one of the healthiest choices of all. It does not only keep you healthy but, also prevents you from getting many dangerous diseases. It helps to lose weight as well as it keeps us healthy strong and fit!

FOUR

HOW TO START A PALEO DIET

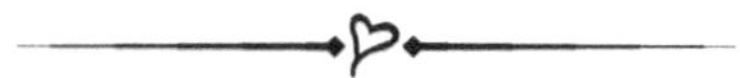

Getting started might not be easy as much as you think. Suddenly, getting used to totally new dietary habits will make you feel pressurized at times. But, this is solely because you are not focused on the great results and also because you haven't started it right.

To have a good continuation and to experience a healthy lifestyle, it is important that you start the Palaeolithic dietary style in a right manner. Here is a step by step guide to tackle the transition;

1. **Get the gut irritating foods out**

Stopping all restricted foods at once might not be practically possible with everyone. Hence doing it in a step by step manner will help you to get used to this new change. Start focusing on gluten first. Take out all gluten containing foods out of your diet; as an example, wheat, oats, barley and even all those glutens hidden ingredients such as malt. But, this doesn't mean that you can eat non-Paleo foods like gluten free breads, rice, etc.

Then slowly start removing all legumes and then the processed foods. Next, move on to dairy products; starting from milk, leave all kinds of butters, creams, ghee and etc.

2. Start cooking at home

This diet needs a lot more attention than you need when you eat junk. It is important that you cook all your food at home, as Paleo foods are very hard to find outside.

Separate a time for cooking and eating, while trying out those easy Paleo recipes once a week. I'm sure you will be surprised to know how tasty Paleo diets can be.

If you are struggling with time management, then try finding an easy Paleo meal plan, which will fit your timetable.

3. Get used to proteins

Paleo diets contain a great amount of proteins and you who have eaten carbs and fats the most have to start getting used to taste the proteins in every single meal. Actually, many people love this change during converting to Paleo. Grilled meat or a baked fish are all that you need when you want to satisfy your taste buds!

4. Time to think about carbohydrates

A Paleo diet is a dairy free diet, but it is not a carb free or low carb diet. It is you, who should focus on keeping the starches low. Some people may add a lot of starchy vegetables in their Paleo diet. But, if you are also focused on losing weight while turning into Paleo then add low carb fruits and veggies to your Paleo diet.

5. **The fats!**

Start using tallow, lard, bacon fat (all preferably pastured), and coconut oil as your main cooking fats. Use olive oil, grape seed oil and macadamia nut oil as your raw fats (like salad dressings). Also, start thinking about your omega-3 to omega-6 intake. For this, you may add enough of large sea fishes to your diet or take some simple supplements. But, I prefer the former.

6. **The food quality is important**

Now that you are Paleo think about the freshness, quality and nutritional value of each and everything you buy. Doing it right and doing it in with high quality, help you get better results.

7. **Clean your pantry**

Now it is the time to throw all unnecessary food stuffs out of your house. The butters the biscuits, snacks, chocolates and etc. should be directly out of your house. This makes you get less tempted and distracted. As I once said, getting used to this new life needs time and your effort and now that you have made your kitchen Paleolithic, it is the time to change the rest of your house as well.

Some say hanging a picture of a Paleo diet in the dining room encourages them to remain Paleo.

8. **Find support**

One of the toughest things about switching to a Paleo diet can be the lack of understanding from friends and family. To co-op with this, find some blogs to read and some forums where you can post questions. See if any of your friends/acquaintances have restricted diets. Feeling like you are part of a Paleo community will help you find ways to cope with questions and uninformed judgments from those around you. Every good change has a criticism after all!!

FIVE

PALEO DIET GUIDELINES

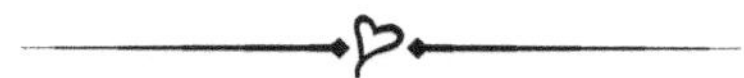

1. A Paleo diet must be high in animal proteins, moderate in good fats and low in carbohydrates. Actually, calorie counting is not encouraged in this diet or the portion control.

2. Eat generous amount of saturated fats such as coconut oil, butter and ghee. Lard, duck fat and tallow are better options for cooking while olive oil, avocado oil, macadamia and grape seed oils are better options for salad dressings.

3. Eat a lot of animal proteins like red meat, poultry, pork and also fishes and sea foods. Also, learn to cook bones in the form of stock and broths.

4. Eat the same amount of fresh or frozen veggies and fruits. Better served them cooked or raw.

5. Eat moderate amounts of fruits and nuts. Try to eat fruits low in sugar and high in vitamins and antioxidants like berries. Nuts, such as almonds, macadamia are better options to fulfil the daily need of omega 3 and omega 6.

6. Preferably choose pastureraised and grass-fed meat from local, environmentally conscious farms. If not possible, choose lean cuts of meat.

7. Stop all cereals, grains and legumes from the diet. This includes wheat, rye, barley, oats, corn, soy, brown rice, peanuts, kidney beans, pinto beans and etc.

8. Cut all vegetable oils which are fully or partially hydrogenated. As an example, they can be sunflower oil, safflower oil, margarine, soya bean oil, canola oil, corn oil and peanut oil.

9. Eliminate all added sugars, starting from refined sugars to all those sweets, juices, soft drinks and snacks.

10. No dairy product should be added to the Paleo diet, as it is a dairy free diet. The Palaeolithic men never knew to grow animals or milk them.

11. Eat when you're hungry and don't stress if you skip a meal or even two. You don't have to eat three square meals a day, do what feels most natural.

12. Consider taking supplements with vitamin D and probiotics. Levels of magnesium, iodine and vitamin K2 should also be optimized. Iodine can be obtained from

seaweeds and sea salts you use.

13. Do not over exercise. Keep your training session in an optimized time scale and over exercising won't get you anywhere. Let the proteins of the Paleo diet help you while the body slowly use the stored fat to be wasted during exercises.

14. Try out new Paleo recipes to encourage your cooking skills as well as taste buds.

15. Play in the sun, have fun, be active, laugh, relax, travel, discover and never hesitate to enjoy life

SIX

No Grains! Why?

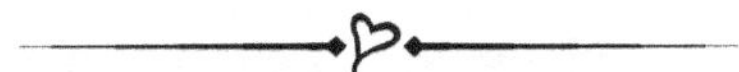

Now you know that grains and legumes are not allowed in Paleo diet as much as the dairy products are as well. It is not only because the Palaeolithic men did not eat them, but, there is also another secret behind it, which we or maybe even the Palaeolithic men did not know.

The pale diet focuses a lot about avoiding gut irritating foods and keeping the omega 3 and omega 6 ration well balanced at the same time. Grains and legumes seem to have negative effects on both of the aspects.

The normal ratio between omega 3 and omega 6 should be 1:1 or 1:2. Grains and legumes are rich in linoleic acids – an omega 6 fatty acid, which in large quantities may cause many diseases in your organism. Omega 6 fatty acids in large quantities contribute to the inflammatory mechanisms in your body and thus, may result in many modern day diseases. This kind of fats are packed in the modern day vegetable oils which are partially or fully hydrogenated; as examples, sunflower oil, safflower oil, margarine, soya been oil, canola oil, corn oil and peanut oil. The oils of grains and legumes were introduced only after the mechanical extraction was invented. Therefore, these fatty acids do not come in only by eating grains and legumes, but, also by consuming their oils. That is why the Paleo diet, says no to these vegetable oils, made out of grains and legumes.

Another way the omega 3: omega 6 balance will break down is when we consume meat of animals that are fed with grains. The meat of these animals contains a ratio of about 1:10. It is not enough just to avoid grains in your diet; you need to be mindful of what you eat that eats grains too. In the modern world, we would eat poultry and meat that have no proper balance between these fatty acids and that is why the Paleo guidelines say, that you should find grass fed and pasture raised animals' meat.

Grains have high concentrations of two types of lectins, which are called as prolamines and agglutinins. These lectins are proteins that supply the natural protection of the plant from predators and pests. They act in the same way in human bodies. Hence, they are of great concern for human health.

These lectins can either damage the cells, lining the gut wall or cause spaces to open up between gut cells. These spaces are like holes and through them substances leak out into the bloodstream. These leaks can let some chemicals of the food mix with blood, and they induce inflammation of tissues and cells.

Among all lectins, the most dangerous has been gluten ad it is known that it takes six months for the gut to get healed after a single gluten exposure.

Lectins also act as anti-nutrients by preventing absorption of many vitamins and minerals in the gut.

Above all grains are highly acidic food in the level of the kidneys. The Palaeolithic diet also concerns about acid-base balance. But, when grains are present in the diet, it is really impossible to neutralize using alkaline foods and this high acidity will strain on the kidneys, liver and pancreas. Therefore, don't you think legumes and grains are a bad choice for a healthy diet?

SEVEN
PALEO FOR KIDS

Many people ask whether the Palaeolithic nutrition is suitable for kids and the answer is – yes, of course. The kids can even benefit more than the adults. Moreover, it is even easier to make this difference, if you start the Paleo diet in the early childhood. This age is the age when children develop their dietary habits, and giving Paleo food at this age will help the kids develop the Palaeolithic dietary habits very easily.

It is a known fact that the need of nutrition is higher in kids than a normal person. It is because they are growing and growing faster. For a healthy and an optimum growth, it is important that these kids get all kinds of nutritional components in the correct amount. The need of Omega 3 is really high in children as the brain development of kids is high at this age. Also, the colourful veggies and fruits are the great sources of vitamins and minerals for the growing children. It is very clear that the Paleo diet is a nutritionally dense diet than any other.

Also, the guts of the kids are not developed completely and the lectins like proteins can damage the gut lining very easily, than in an adult.

If you just had a child, and thinking of changing to Paleo, definitely this is the perfect time. Avocado, banana, sweet potato, squash, applesauce and egg yolk are excellent options as first food. If you give Paleo food from the beginning, it will be easy for you to bring the child up with Palaeolithic dietary habits. But, if you have an older child and going to make this change, you will have to go through some difficulties. Many kids are picky and crave all those junk foods. But remember, any improvement to your kid's nutrition worth all the frustration, so keep trying.

It is okay if your child is not perfectly Paleo. A child needs a lot of carbohydrates as they are highly active. But, always remember to fulfil this energy need with natural carbohydrates and fats. Anyhow, the refined sugars, processed foods and other sweets should be eliminated from the diet. Moreover, there will be circumstances when you will have to go out of the tract; especially, when your kid has birthday parties and other celebrations. Therefore, let's not make a big deal out of those occasional treats, but also strive toward a tasty, healthy variety of Paleo foods at home.

Then what about dairy? This is the trick here. It is well known that dairy proteins and calcium are necessary for child development at least until the age of 5. In the Palaeolithic era, this was fulfilled by breastfeeding kids until they are old enough. But, new researches show that the quality of breast milk reduces after 9 months from birth, hence, it is important to give the kids dairy. This addition of milk products to a Paleo meal is known as lacto-Paleo diet or primal diet.

To avoid the gut irritating chemicals in commercial dairy products in the market, try to stick into the cultured dairy products such as yoghurt, curd, kefir. It is even better if you can find fresh milk from grass-fed cows of the local farmers. Goat's milk and goat's milk products are also a good choice because they tend to be less problematic, and are very easy to find these days.

But, remember soy milk is not a correct substitute for cow's milk even for kids. Legumes are strictly avoided in Paleo diet and the additions of milk and dairy in lacto Paleo diets should only be of animal origin.

Now that you know how to optimize your Paleo diet for your kids, you may easily change your whole family into Paleo. Starting from your parents to your kids, you know what to let them eat. Get a good Paleo recipe book and surprise your family with the extraordinarily healthy and tasty meals.

EIGHT

GRAY AREA FOODS

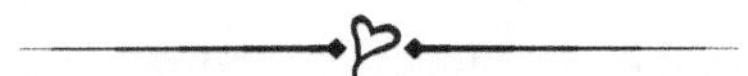

The Paleo diet focuses not only on avoiding gut irritating foods but also of preventing insulin resistance and hormonal imbalances. But, there are some foods which are in the middle of should and should not's and they are called gray area foods. Actually, it is controversial whether they are safe or not. It is you who should choose whether to include them in your diet or not.

Many Paleo specialists suggest that you cut off these foods from your Paleo diet for about a month or two and then slowly adding them back, one at a time to see how they make you feel.

Here are the main gray area foods;

- Nuts and seeds

Nuts and seeds contain small amounts of gut irritating foods and anti-nutrients. You can reduce these chemicals by soaking them in water.

- Nightshades

Veggie such as peppers, eggplant, tomatoes and potatoes contain small amounts of toxic chemicals. Depending on your body's capabilities you may or may not be sensitive to these chemicals. A better option is to eat the ripest version of these veggies. When it comes to potatoes, peeling them off reduces these toxic substances.

- Eggs

Eggs can make problems for some people as well. A chemical called lysozyme can let your gut leak substances into your bloodstream. According to the findings, the egg yolk is the healthier part of an egg. Isn't that strange?

- Coffee

You know that coffee contains caffeine. Coffee and caffeinated beverages increase the Cortisol hormone level in your blood. Cortisol hormone is known to be a stress hormone, which is normally produced by the adrenal glands when the mind or body is in stress. This stress hormone changes many physiological activities in the body, which in the long run may result in various disorders. Today, we are more focused on reducing stress, but, caffeine may totally do the opposite of it.

- Alcohol

The problem with alcohol is the dose. A small quantity about 6-12 oz a day helps in preventing heart diseases while more than that will result in heart attacks and strokes.

Alcohol is not prohibited in Paleo diet. But, you should watch out on how much you take.

A glass of red wine can be good and a healthy option with a tasty Paleo meal. But, don't get fooled by the tasty beers which contain malt and glutens.

With all gray area foods, it is better to consider them as culprits and avoid. If you cannot avoid, then reduce the quantity and frequency you use them.

Going Paleo is all about having a healthy life, then why do we have to be misled by even one of our craves?

NINE

What You Should Eat

Meat	Fish	Sea Food
Poultry	Bass	Crab
Turkey	Salmon	Crawfish
Chicken Pork tenderloin	Halibut	Crayfish
Pork chops	Mackerel	Shrimp
Steak	Sardines	Clams
Veal	Tuna	Lobster
Bacon	Red snapper	Scallops
Pork	Shark	Oysters
Ground beef	Sunfish	
Grass-fed beef	Swordfish	
Lamb rack	Tilapia	
Shrimp	Trout	
Lobster	Walleye	
Clams		
Salmon		
Venison steaks		
Buffalo		

New York steak		
Bison		
Lamb chops		
Rabbit		
Goat		
Elk		
Emu		
Goose		
Kangaroo		
Bear		
Beef jerky		
Eggs		
Wild boar		
Reindeer		
Turtle		
Ostrich		
Pheasant		
Quail		
Lean veal		
Chuck steak		
Rattlesnake		

vegetables	Fats/oils
Asparagus	Coconut oil
Avocado	Olive oil
Artichoke hearts	Macadamia oil
Brussels sprouts	Avocado oil
Carrots	
Spinach	
Celery	
Broccoli	
Zucchini	
Cabbage	
Peppers (all kinds)	
Cauliflower	
Parsley	
Eggplant	
Green onions	
Butternut squash	
Acorn squash	
Yam	
Sweet potato	
Beets	

Nuts	Fruits
Almonds	Apple
Cashews	Avocado
Hazelnuts	Blackberries
Pecans	Papaya
Pine nuts	Peaches
Pumpkin seeds	Plums
Sunflower seeds	Mango

Macadamia nuts	Lychee
Walnuts	Blueberries
	Grapes
	Lemon
	Strawberries
	Watermelon
	Pineapple guava
	Lime
	Raspberries
	Cantaloupe
	Tangerine
	Figs
	Oranges
	Bananas

TEN

WHAT YOU SHOULD NOT EAT

Dairy	Drinks	Grains
Butter	Coke, Sprite, Pepsi	Cereals
Cheese	Mountain Dew etc.	Bread, Toast
Non-fat dairy creamer	Juices	English muffins
Milk	Chinola juice	Sandwiches
Dairy spreads	Starfruit juice	Triscuits
Cream cheese	Mango juice	Wheat Thins
Powdered milk	Red Bull, Monster	Crackers, Oatmeal
Yogurt	Rockstar	Cream of wheat
Pudding	Starbucks Refreshers	Corn, Corn syrup
Frozen yogurt	Mountain Dew MDX	High-fructose corn syrup
Ice milk	Vault, XS Energy Drink	Wheat, Pancakes
Low-fat milk	5-Hour Energy	Hash browns
Ice cream		Beer (and the world mourned)
		Pasta

Legumes	Others
Black beans	Artificial sweeteners
Broad beans	Alcohols
Fava beans	Snacks
Garbanzo beans	Sweets
Horse beans	Salty foods
Kidney beans	
Lima beans	
Mung beans	
Adzuki beans	
Navy beans	
Pinto beans	
Black-eyed peas (and, yes, you should also avoid the band)	
Chickpeas	
Snowpeas	
Sugar snap peas	
Peanuts	
Peanut butter	
Miso	
Lentils	
Lupins	
Mesquite	
Soybeans	
All soybean products and derivatives	
Tofu	
Any other beans.	

ELEVEN

PALEO MEAL PLAN

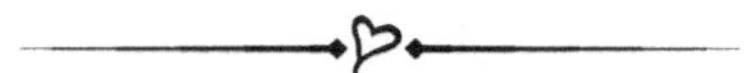

As in normal diet plans, a Paleo diet plan should consist of 3 main meals and 2 snacks. But, all meals and snacks should be Paleo friendly. It is not necessary that you eat all five times. Adjust it in a way which is comfortable for you.

Here is a simple example of a Paleo meal plan.

Breakfast: Scrambled eggs with smoked salmon

Snack 01:3-4 Papaya slices

Lunch: Salad with roast chicken, dried cranberries, pecans, apple slices, and vinaigrette.

Snack 02: Handful of nuts or trail mix

Dinner: Ham and Pineapple Skewers with oven-roasted tomatoes.

TWELVE
RECIPES

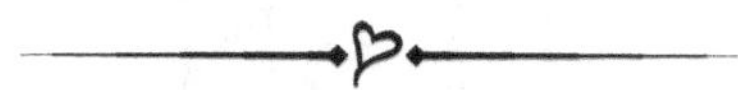

Chinese-style green beans.

Ingredients:

- 250 gm lean bacon, cut into pieces
- 400 gm beans, slice diagonally into strip
- 1 onion chopped
- 1 garlic clove. Chopped
- 2 tablespoons olive oil
- 2 tablespoons soy sauce

Method:

1. Bean strips cook in a steamer until tender.
2. Fry onion, garlic in olive oil, add bacon and cook until pale gold.
3. Steamed bean strips return to pan.
4. Stir in bacon mixture and soy sauce heat gently shaking pan.

Chicken & bell pepper fry in Iceberg.

Ingredients:

- 500 gm chicken breast cut into strips
- 3 yellow bell pepper, seeded and sliced into strip
- 1 onion sliced
- 1 tablespoons olive oil
- 1 tsp orange peel
- ½ cup orange juice
- 3 cloves garlic, chopped
- 1 tsp ginger, chopped
- 1 cup almond, coarsely chopped
- ½ cup green scallions, sliced
- 8-10 Iceberg lettuces

Method:

1. In pan heat the olive oil, add chicken cook for 2 -3 minutes.
2. Add bell pepper, onion and cook for another 2-3 minutes.
3. Remove the mixture from pan and keep aside.
4. Add orange juice into pan cook 3 minutes to boil.
5. Add ginger, garlic, and cook another 1 minute.
6. Return the chicken & bell pepper mixture to the pan
7. Stir in orange peel, almond & scallion
8. Stir-fry on Iceberg lettuces.

Fruity Kebabs.

Ingredients:

- 1 red Apple cut into pieces
- ½ pineapples cut into pieces
- 200 gm strawberries washed
- ½ lemon juice
- 2 mango cut into pieces
- 1 cup low fat yogurt

Method:

1. Brush Apple with lemon juice.
2. Thread pineapple, Red apple, Mango & strawberries onto kebab sticks.
3. Dip into yogurt & serve.

Chicken with Avocado

Ingredients:

- 1 large chicken breast
- 1 cup chicken broth
- 1 large tomato diced
- 1 tablespoon tomato paste
- 1 Jalepenos.de seeded & diced
- 1 onion diced
- 1 large carrot, shredded
- 1 bunch coriander leaves, chopped
- 2 tablespoon olive oil
- 2 clove garlic, chopped
- ½ tsp chili powder
- ½ tsp cumin
- Salt & pepper
- 2 Avocados

- 1 cup water

Method:

1. In a pan heat the olive oil.
2. Add onions, garlic
3. Add ¼ cup chicken broth.
4. Add salt, pepper.
5. Then add chicken Brest and remaining ingredients (without avocado & coriander leaves).
6. Add enough water to cover the chicken Brest
7. Add salt & pepper needed
8. Let cook on slow fire about30minutes.
9. Chicken is well-cooked break the chicken apart & into shred.
10. Top avocado slices & fresh chopped coriander leaves.

Beef cakes with Mushroom sauce

<u>Beef cake</u>
Ingredients:

- 250 gm Beef boil & mince
- 1 large onion, chopped
- 1 clove garlic, chopped
- 1 tablespoon salary, chopped
- ½ tsp oregano
- ½ tsp mixed herbs
- 1 egg
- 2 tablespoon olive oil
- Salt & pepper

Method:

1. Mix minced beef, onion, garlic, salary, egg, oregano, mixed herbs all together.
2. Mix well with salt & pepper to taste.
3. Make flat balls.
4. In the pan heat olive oil and add the chicken balls and cook until golden brown on each side.

<u>Mushroom sauce</u>
Ingredients:

- 2 tablespoon butter.
- 50 gm mushroom
- 1 tomato
- ½ tablespoon chopped salary
- 1 tsp soy sauce
- 1 tablespoon vinegar
- ½ cup water
- Salt, Pepper

Method:

1. In pan heat the butter
2. Add sliced mushrooms, cook until soft.
3. Add water, peeled and chopped tomatoes, vinegar.
4. Add soy sauce and stir until sauce thickens.
5. Add salary, salt& pepper.
6. At last pour sauce onto beef cakes.

Disclaimer

Introduction

By using this book, you accept this disclaimer in full.

No advice

The book contains information. The information is not advice and should not be treated as such.

No representations or warranties

To the maximum extent permitted by applicable law and subject to section below, we exclude all representations, warranties, undertakings and guarantees relating to the book.

Without prejudice to the generality of the foregoing paragraph, we do not represent, warrant, undertake or guarantee:

- that the information in the book is correct, accurate, complete or non-misleading.

- that the use of the guidance in the book will lead to any particular outcome or result.

Limitations and exclusions of liability

The limitations and exclusions of liability set out in this section and elsewhere in this disclaimer: are subject to section 6 below; and govern all liabilities arising under the disclaimer or in relation to the book, including liabilities arising in contract, in tort (including negligence) and for breach of statutory duty.

We will not be liable to you in respect of any losses arising out of any event or events beyond our reasonable control.

We will not be liable to you in respect of any business losses, including without limitation loss of or damage to profits, income, revenue, use, production, anticipated savings, business, contracts, commercial opportunities or goodwill.

We will not be liable to you in respect of any loss or corruption of any data, database or software.

We will not be liable to you in respect of any special, indirect or consequential loss or damage.

Exceptions

Nothing in this disclaimer shall: limit or exclude our liability for death or personal injury resulting from negligence; limit or exclude our liability for fraud or fraudulent misrepresentation; limit any of our liabilities in any way that is not permitted under applicable law; or exclude any of our liabilities that may not be excluded under applicable law.

Severability

If a section of this disclaimer is determined by any court or other competent authority to be unlawful and/or unenforceable, the other sections of this disclaimer continue in effect.

If any unlawful and/or unenforceable section would be lawful or enforceable if part of it were deleted, that part will be deemed to be deleted, and the rest of the section will continue in effect.

Law and jurisdiction

This disclaimer will be governed by and construed in accordance with Swiss law, and any disputes relating to this disclaimer will be subject to the exclusive jurisdiction of the courts of Switzerland.